HOW TO PREVENT GALLSTONES COOKBOOK

Essential Recipes for Healthy and Delicious Meals to Protect Your Gallbladder and Improve Digestive Health

DR LANA BROWN, RN

Copyright Page

© 2024 by Dr. Lana Brown.

All rights reserved. No part of this cookbook may be reproduced, distributed, or transmitted in any form or by any means, including photocopying, recording, or other electronic or mechanical methods, without the prior written permission of the author, except in the case of brief quotations embodied in critical reviews and certain other noncommercial uses permitted by copyright law.

For permissions requests, write to the author at www.thelanabrown.com

Table of Contents

Copyright Page 2

Table of Contents 3

INTRODUCTION 1

WHAT ARE GALLSTONES? 4

    Causes Symptoms and Complications 7

    The Importance of Prevention 11

THE SCIENCE BEHIND GALLSTONES 12

    Formation of Gallstones 13

    Types of Gallstones 13

    Risk Factors and Triggers 15

    Dietary Habits 17

WHY PREVENT GALLSTONES? 19

    The Role of Diet in Prevention 20

    Recognizing Early Symptoms 21

PRINCIPLES OF A GALLSTONE PREVENTION DIET 23

Foods to Include 24

Foods to Avoid 25

Sample Meal Plan for Gallstone Prevention 26

NOURISHING BREAKFAST RECIPES FOR GALLSTONE PREVENTION 28

Baked Oatmeal Cups 28

Fiesta Tofu Scramble 30

Fire Avocado Toast 33

Omelette 34

Microwaved "Fried" Rice 36

Apple Slices 38

Caprese Avocado Toast 39

Low-Carb Blueberry Muffins 41

Date & Pine Nut Overnight Oatmeal 43

Bagel Avocado Toast 44

Baked Banana-Nut Oatmeal Cups 45

Pineapple Green Smoothie 47

Muesli with Raspberries 48

NOURISHING LUNCH RECIPES FOR GALLSTONE PREVENTION 49

Butternut squash and sweet potato soup 49

Crunchy nachos with avocado dip 52

Carrot and Coriander Soup 55

Tomato Watercress Bruschetta 57

Falafel with aubergine dip 59

Mediterranean Chicken Bagel 62

Butter Bean and Sundried Tomato Dip 64

Veggie Burgers 66

Shakshuka with Garlic Pittas 69

Mediterranean Soup 73

NOURISHING DINNER RECIPES FOR GALLSTONE PREVENTION 76

Savory Chicken kebabs with garlic sauce and pickles 76

Savory Veggie Lasagne 79

Tuna Pasta Bake 82

Plaice goujons with a California Walnut Crust 85

Prawn and Vegetable Curry 87

Savory Chinese Chicken Curry 90

Sardines and Pasta 92

Sea Bass with a Vegetable Ensemble 95

Savory Prawn skewers with flatbreads 99

Savory Roasted tomato and broccoli pasta 101

Spanish Fish Stew 105

Savory Spicy Burgers 108

NOURISHING MAIN DISH RECIPES FOR GALLSTONE PREVENTION 110

- Chipotle Black Bean Chili 110
- Okra and Octopus Pasta Bowl 113
- Chicken Biryani 116
- Black Beans and Rice 119
- Pesto Pasta with Chicken 121

NOURISHING SOUP RECIPES FOR GALLSTONE PREVENTION 123

- Red Lentil Dhal Soup with Indian Spiced Broccoli 123
- Pea and Edamame Soup 127
- Spiced Lentil and Carrot Soup 128
- Mushroom and Hazelnut Broth 130
- Barley and Mushroom Chicken Soup 132
- Chunky Tomato Basil Sauce 134

Walk Away Slow-Cook Chicken 136

Southern Fish Stew 137

BEFORE YOU LEAVE, A FINAL WORD!............141

INTRODUCTION

Gallstones are solid particles that form from digestive fluids in your gallbladder. This small, pear-shaped organ is located on the right side of your abdomen, just under your liver. The gallbladder's main function is to store bile, a digestive fluid produced by your liver, and release it into your small intestine when you eat.

While some gallstones cause no symptoms and don't need treatment, others can cause significant discomfort and may require the removal of the gallbladder. Symptoms occur when gallstones block the ducts that move bile from the gallbladder to the small intestine. These symptoms can include sudden, intense pain in the upper right part of the abdomen, rapidly increasing pain in the center of the abdomen below the breastbone, pain between the shoulder blades or in the right shoulder, and nausea or vomiting.

Gallstone pain can last from a few minutes to several hours. If you experience any of these symptoms, it's important to consult with your doctor. Immediate medical attention is needed if you experience severe abdominal pain, jaundice (yellowing of the skin and eyes), or a high fever with chills, as these could be signs of serious complications.

Gallstones can vary greatly in size, ranging from tiny grains of sand to as large as golf balls. Some people may have just one gallstone, while others can develop multiple at the same time.

CHAPTER I
WHAT ARE GALLSTONES?

Gallstones, known medically as cholelithiasis, are hard, pebble-like masses that form in the gallbladder. This small, pear-shaped organ is located on the right side of your abdomen, just below your liver. Gallstones can vary significantly in size, from as tiny as a grain of sand to as large as a golf ball. They can be made of undissolved cholesterol, termed cholesterol gallstones, or the digestive fluid bile, known as pigment gallstones. You might develop a single gallstone or multiple ones simultaneously.

One of the main complications of gallstones is that they can block the tubes, or ducts, that transport digestive fluids from the gallbladder to the bowel. This blockage can cause significant pain and other distressing symptoms. Understanding the role of diet in the prevention of gallstones is crucial for maintaining gallbladder health and avoiding these painful episodes.

The gallbladder plays an essential role in the digestive process by storing and releasing bile, a fluid produced by the liver to help digest fats. When there is an imbalance in the substances that make up bile, such as cholesterol and bilirubin, gallstones can form. Therefore, a diet aimed at preventing gallstones focuses on maintaining this delicate balance and supporting overall digestive health.

Dietary choices are vital in keeping the gallbladder functioning correctly and preventing the formation of gallstones. By carefully selecting foods that promote a healthy balance of cholesterol and bile, individuals can significantly reduce their risk of developing gallstones. This approach not only helps in preventing the formation of new stones but also in managing existing ones to avoid complications.

Understanding the connection between diet and gallstone formation is the first step toward effective prevention. Through mindful eating and making the right nutritional choices, it is possible to support your gallbladder's health and reduce the risk of gallstones, thus ensuring smoother and pain-free digestion.

Causes Symptoms and Complications

Gallstones form due to various imbalances in the bile within the gallbladder. One major cause is an excess of cholesterol. Under normal conditions, bile helps dissolve cholesterol produced by the liver. However, if the liver produces more cholesterol than the bile can manage, it leads to the formation of cholesterol gallstones, which are typically yellow in color.

Another factor is an overproduction of bilirubin, a substance produced from the breakdown of red blood cells. Conditions such as liver damage, infections, or blood disorders can lead to an excess of bilirubin. When the gallbladder cannot process this excess bilirubin, it results in the formation of dark brown or black pigment gallstones.

Inadequate emptying of the gallbladder also contributes to gallstone formation. The gallbladder must regularly empty bile to prevent it from becoming concentrated and forming stones. When this process is impaired, it can lead to the development of gallstones.

Symptoms

Gallstones are often asymptomatic, meaning they may not cause noticeable issues. When symptoms do occur, they typically involve pain in the upper right abdomen. This pain can be triggered by eating fatty, spicy, or fried foods. It may also radiate to the center of the abdomen, just below the breastbone, or even the shoulder blades.

Other symptoms associated with gallstones include nausea, vomiting, diarrhea, and indigestion. These symptoms often accompany the pain and indicate that the gallstones are causing digestive disturbances.

Complications

Complications from gallstones can be severe, particularly if the stones become large or block bile ducts. One serious complication is cholecystitis, which is inflammation of the gallbladder caused by a gallstone obstructing its neck. This can result in intense pain and fever.

Gallstones may also block the common bile duct, leading to an excess concentration of bile in the gallbladder. Similarly, if gallstones obstruct the pancreatic duct, it can impede digestion by preventing pancreatic juices from flowing properly.

In rare cases, a family history of gallstones may increase the risk of gallbladder cancer. Untreated gallstones can also lead to other complications such as infections of the gallbladder or bile ducts, jaundice, sepsis (a severe blood infection), and pancreatic inflammation. Addressing these complications typically requires prompt medical intervention to prevent more severe health problems.

The Importance of Prevention

Preventing gallstones is crucial for maintaining overall health and avoiding the discomfort and potential complications associated with them. By understanding the causes and symptoms of gallstones, individuals can make informed decisions about their diet and lifestyle. Adopting a preventive approach can significantly reduce the risk of gallstone formation and promote better digestive health. Making mindful dietary choices, such as reducing intake of high-cholesterol and fatty foods, increasing fiber intake, and maintaining a healthy weight, can help prevent the development of gallstones and contribute to overall well-being.

CHAPTER II
THE SCIENCE BEHIND GALLSTONES

Gallstones are hard, pebble-like masses that form in the gallbladder, a small organ located on the right side of the abdomen, beneath the liver. The gallbladder stores bile, a digestive fluid produced by the liver. Gallstones can develop when the substances that make up bile—cholesterol and bilirubin—become imbalanced and form solid particles.

Formation of Gallstones

Gallstones form when there is an imbalance in the composition of bile. When the liver produces too much cholesterol or bilirubin, or when the gallbladder does not empty efficiently, these substances can crystallize and form stones. Cholesterol gallstones, the most common type, occur when there is too much cholesterol in the bile. Pigment gallstones form when there is excess bilirubin, often due to liver damage or blood disorders.

Types of Gallstones

There are two main types of gallstones:

Cholesterol Gallstones: These are usually yellow-green and primarily composed of undissolved cholesterol. They are the most common type, accounting for about 80% of gallstones.

Cholesterol gallstones are the most common type, accounting for about 75% of all gallstones. These stones are primarily composed of cholesterol, a fatty substance found in bile. They form when there is an excess of cholesterol in the bile or when the gallbladder does not empty efficiently. Cholesterol gallstones are typically yellow-green in color and can vary significantly in size.

Pigment Gallstones: These stones are dark brown or black and are made of bilirubin. They tend to form in individuals with liver disease or blood disorders.

Pigment gallstones account for the remaining 20% to 25% of gallstone cases. These stones are made of bilirubin, a pigment formed from the breakdown of red blood cells. Pigment gallstones are usually smaller and darker, ranging in color from brown to black. They commonly occur in individuals with certain medical conditions, such as cirrhosis, hemolytic anemia, or specific infections.

Risk Factors and Triggers

Several factors can increase the risk of developing gallstones, including:

- Obesity: Excess body weight increases cholesterol levels in bile and decreases gallbladder emptying.
- Rapid Weight Loss: Losing weight quickly can cause the liver to secrete extra cholesterol into bile.

- Diet: High-fat, high-cholesterol, and low-fiber diets can contribute to gallstone formation.
- Gender and Age: Women and individuals over 40 are at higher risk.
- Ethnicity: Native American and Mexican American populations have a higher prevalence of gallstones.
- Medical Conditions: Diabetes, liver disease, and certain gastrointestinal diseases can increase risk.
- Hormones: High estrogen levels from pregnancy, hormone replacement therapy, or birth control pills can raise the risk.
- Genetics: A family history of gallstones increases the likelihood of developing them.

Dietary Habits

To reduce the risk of gallstones, consider adopting the following dietary habits:

- Don't Skip Meals: Skipping meals or fasting can increase the risk of gallstones. Maintain regular meal times to ensure the gallbladder empties frequently.
- Lose Weight Slowly: Aim for gradual weight loss, about 1-2 pounds per week, to avoid triggering gallstone formation.
- Eat High-Fiber Foods: Incorporate plenty of fruits, vegetables, and whole grains into your diet to help maintain a healthy digestive system.
- Maintain a Healthy Weight: Achieving and maintaining a healthy weight reduces the risk of gallstones. Balance your caloric intake with regular physical activity.

- Stay Hydrated: Drink enough water each day to support digestive health.
- Eat Smaller, Frequent Meals: Smaller, more frequent meals can help keep bile flowing and prevent gallstones.

CHAPTER III

WHY PREVENT GALLSTONES?

Preventing gallstones is essential to avoid the pain and complications associated with these stones. While it's not possible to guarantee complete prevention, adopting healthy dietary and lifestyle habits can significantly reduce the risk. This includes maintaining a healthy weight, eating a balanced diet rich in fiber, staying hydrated, and avoiding rapid weight loss strategies. Regular exercise and not skipping meals are also important preventive measures. If you have specific concerns or a family history of gallstones, consult with your healthcare provider for personalized advice and guidance.

The Role of Diet in Prevention

Diet plays a crucial role in preventing gallstones. While there's no proven way to prevent them entirely, maintaining a well-balanced diet, a normal weight, and regular exercise are key strategies. Avoiding foods high in saturated fats and refined carbohydrates can help reduce the risk of gallstone formation. Instead, focus on a diet rich in whole grains, vegetables, and fruits, which helps keep bile cholesterol in liquid form and supports overall gallbladder health. Consuming healthy fats like fish oil and olive oil in moderation can also aid in regular gallbladder contraction and bile emptying. However, it's important not to cut out fats abruptly, as too little fat can also lead to gallstone formation.

Recognizing Early Symptoms

Recognizing the early symptoms of gallstones is crucial for timely intervention and treatment. A stone lodged in a duct can lead to more serious problems, such as acute cholecystitis (inflammation of the gallbladder), pancreatitis (inflammation of the pancreas), or cholangitis (inflammation of the bile ducts in the liver). These conditions can cause severe pain, jaundice, high fever, chills, and vomiting, often requiring hospitalization and surgical removal of the stone. If you experience sudden and severe pain that lasts for hours, it's important to seek medical help immediately. Diagnostic tests like blood tests, abdominal ultrasound, cholescintigraphy, MRI, endoscopic ultrasonography, and endoscopic retrograde cholangiopancreatography can help identify the presence and severity of gallstones and guide appropriate treatment.

By understanding the importance of a gallstone prevention diet and recognizing the early symptoms of gallstones, you can take proactive steps to maintain your gallbladder health and avoid the painful and potentially serious complications associated with this condition.

CHAPTER IV
PRINCIPLES OF A GALLSTONE PREVENTION DIET

A gallstone prevention diet focuses on reducing the risk of gallstones and managing symptoms if they develop. Gallstones, or cholelithiasis, are formed primarily from cholesterol in bile, which can crystallize and create stones. To prevent their formation and reduce complications like gallbladder attacks and inflammation, certain dietary principles should be followed.

Foods to Include

In contrast, certain foods can help prevent gallstones and support gallbladder health. Fruits are beneficial as they contain little fat and allow the gallbladder to rest. Regular consumption of fruits like apples and pears can help make bile more fluid, reducing the risk of stone formation. Legumes, high in fiber and low in fat, have been shown to lower the risk of gallstones. Artichokes are particularly useful as they help make bile more fluid and support gallbladder emptying, reducing the risk of sediment and stone formation. Similarly, radishes and soy products, including soy milk and tofu, can enhance bile production and reduce cholesterol levels, which may help prevent stones.

Foods rich in fiber, such as whole grains, fruits, and vegetables, are essential as they help maintain regular bile flow and prevent stone formation. Vitamin C is also beneficial; studies have shown that a higher intake of vitamin C can reduce the risk of gallstones. Lastly, lecithin, found in soy products and nuts, helps improve cholesterol solubility in bile, preventing stone formation.

Foods to Avoid

To prevent gallstones, it is crucial to avoid foods that can exacerbate the condition. High-fat foods, such as fried items (e.g., fried chicken, French fries) and fatty meats (e.g., beef, pork), can trigger gallbladder contractions, potentially leading to pain and complications.

Dairy products, particularly high-fat varieties like whole milk, cream, and butter, should also be avoided as they can provoke gallbladder contractions and discomfort. Excessive sugars and refined carbohydrates, found in sweets and pastries, can promote gallstone formation. Additionally, processed meats and alcohol should be limited or avoided due to their adverse effects on gallbladder health.

Sample Meal Plan for Gallstone Prevention

Here is a sample meal plan to guide you in incorporating gallstone prevention foods into your diet:

Breakfast: A smoothie made with spinach, a banana, and a handful of berries. Add a tablespoon of chia seeds for extra fiber.

Lunch: A salad with mixed greens, cherry tomatoes, cucumber, chickpeas, and a dressing made with olive oil and lemon juice. Include a side of whole-grain bread.

Snack: An apple or a serving of fresh fruit with a handful of almonds.

Dinner: Grilled salmon with a side of quinoa and steamed broccoli. Finish with a small serving of a citrus fruit like kiwi or orange.

By following these dietary guidelines and incorporating the recommended foods into your meals, you can reduce the risk of gallstones and support overall gallbladder health.

CHAPTER V

NOURISHING BREAKFAST RECIPES FOR GALLSTONE PREVENTION

Baked Oatmeal Cups

INGREDIENTS

for 12 cups

nonstick cooking spray, for greasing

1 ½ cups milk(360 mL)

½ cup applesauce(125 g)

¼ cup nut or sunflower butter(60 g)

¼ cup maple syrup(55 g)

2 teaspoons vanilla extract

2 large eggs

3 cups old-fashioned oats (300 g)

1 teaspoon baking powder

½ teaspoon kosher salt

1 teaspoon ground cinnamon

topping of choice

INSTRUCTIONS

Preheat the oven to 350°F (180°C). Grease a muffin tin with nonstick spray.

Add the milk, applesauce, nut butter, maple syrup, vanilla, and eggs to a medium bowl and whisk until combined.

Add the oats, baking powder, salt, and cinnamon. Stir quickly to make sure everything is well-hydrated.

Divide the batter between the prepared muffin cups, then add your toppings of choice. Bake for 20–25 minutes or until the centers of the muffins spring back when gently pressed.

The oatmeal cups can be enjoyed immediately, or cooled and frozen in an airtight container for up to 2 months. To reheat, microwave for 2 minutes.

Fiesta Tofu Scramble

INGREDIENTS

for 4 servings

1 tablespoon extra virgin olive oil

1 red bell pepper, seeded and diced

1 jalapeño, seeded and diced

¼ medium red onion, diced

kosher salt, to taste

14 oz extra firm tofu(395 g), drained and patted dry

½ teaspoon ground turmeric

1 teaspoon garlic powder

½ teaspoon onion powder

pepper, to taste

¼ cup fresh cilantro leaves(10 g)

½ avocado, sliced

Lime wedge, for garnish

INSTRUCTIONS

Heat the olive oil in a large skillet over medium heat. When the oil is shimmering, add the bell pepper, jalapeño, and red onion. Season with salt. Sauté for 2 minutes, until the vegetables start to sweat.

Crumble the tofu into the pan and stir to break up. Add the turmeric, garlic powder, onion powder, and pepper and stir to combine. Make sure the turmeric evenly coats the tofu to give it an egg-like color.

Serve hot with cilantro, sliced avocado, and lime wedges.

Fire Avocado Toast

INGREDIENTS

for 1 serving

½ avocado

kosher salt, to taste

½ teaspoon hot sauce

1 slice multigrain toast

½ teaspoon red pepper flakes

1 egg, sunny-side up

INSTRUCTIONS

Scoop the avocado into a medium bowl. Season with salt and add the tabasco. Mash until smooth.

Spread the avocado on the slice of toast. Sprinkle with the red pepper flakes and top with the fried egg.

Omelette

INGREDIENTS

for 2 servings

2 tablespoons oil

½ cup ham(75 g), chopped

2 bell peppers, diced

1 cup spinach(40 g)

salt, to taste

pepper, to taste

4 eggs

½ cup jack cheese(65 g), shredded

½ cup shredded cheddar cheese(50 g)

1 avocado, sliced

INSTRUCTIONS

Heat oil in a pan over high heat.

Cook the ham, peppers, and spinach with a pinch of salt and pepper until the spinach has wilted. Transfer to a bowl.

Whisk the 4 eggs with a pinch of salt & pepper, then pour half of the mixture into the pan, swirling it around to make a full circle. Lower to a medium heat.

Cook for about 15 seconds, then spoon half of the veggie mixture on one half of the omelette and sprinkle half of the jack and half the cheddar cheese on the other half.

Cook until the cheese is half melted, then fold one half of the omelette over the other.

Cook for another 15 seconds, then remove and transfer to a plate.

Fan out half of the avocado slices on top of the omelette, then repeat with the other omelette.

Microwaved "Fried" Rice

INGREDIENTS

for 1 serving

½ cup rice(100 g)

2 cups water(480 mL)

1 tablespoon soy sauce

1 teaspoon sesame oil

½ cup frozen vegetable(75 g)

2 eggs

salt, to taste

1 tablespoon scallion, chopped, to serve

INSTRUCTIONS

In a bowl, combine the rice, water, sesame oil, and soy sauce.

Stir, then microwave, covered, for approximately 6-8 minutes until the rice is fully cooked.

Mix the frozen vegetables into the rice.

In a microwaveable mug, beat the eggs.

Microwave the eggs and the rice again for approximately 1-2 minutes, until the eggs are fully cooked.

Break up the egg into small bits, then mix it in with the rice.

Top with scallions, and serve.

Apple Slices

INGREDIENTS

for 1 serving

1 apple

peanut butter, to taste

granola, to taste

1 cup dark chocolate chips(175 g), optional

INSTRUCTIONS

Slice apples horizontally, about ¼-inch (6 ½ mm) thick.

Using a spoon or small round object carefully push the center of the apple out.

Spread on peanut butter, then top with granola and chocolate chips.

Caprese Avocado Toast

INGREDIENTS

for 1 serving

bread, toasted

½ avocado, mashed

salt, to taste

pepper, to taste

2 heirloom tomatoes, sliced

1 mozzarella ball, sliced

1 handful fresh basil, chopped

INSTRUCTIONS

Mash half of an avocado. Add salt and pepper, to taste. Mix until well combined.

Spread the mashed avocado evenly across toast, and top with heirloom tomatoes, mozzarella, and chopped basil.

Low-Carb Blueberry Muffins

INGREDIENTS

1 ¾ cups almond flour

¼ cup coconut flour

1 tablespoon baking powder

¼ teaspoon baking soda

¼ teaspoon salt

1 cup blueberries

3 large eggs

½ cup reduced-fat milk

⅓ cup plus 2 tablespoons light brown sugar

¼ cup avocado oil

1 ½ teaspoons vanilla extract

INSTRUCTIONS

Preheat oven to 350 degrees F. Generously coat a muffin tin with cooking spray.

Sift almond flour, coconut flour, baking powder, baking soda and salt together in a large bowl. Add blueberries and toss to coat. Whisk eggs, milk, brown sugar, oil and vanilla in a medium bowl. Add to the dry ingredients and stir until combined. Divide the batter among the muffin cups (about 1/4 cup batter per cup).

Bake the muffins until lightly browned around the edges and a toothpick inserted in the center comes out clean, 20 to 25 minutes. Let cool in the pan on a wire rack for 20 minutes. Run a knife around the edges and remove from the tin to cool completely.

Date & Pine Nut Overnight Oatmeal

INGREDIENTS

½ cup old-fashioned rolled oats

½ cup water

Pinch of salt

2 tablespoons chopped dates

1 tablespoon toasted pine nuts

1 teaspoon honey

¼ teaspoon ground cinnamon

INSTRUCTIONS

Combine oats, water and salt in a jar or bowl and stir. Cover and refrigerate overnight.

In the morning, heat the oats, if desired, or eat cold. Top with dates, pine nuts, honey and cinnamon.

Tips

Tip: People with celiac disease or gluten sensitivity should use oats that are labeled "gluten-free," as oats are often cross-contaminated with wheat and barley.

To make ahead: When prepping oatmeal the night before, measure, toast and chop ingredients for the topping.

Bagel Avocado Toast

INGREDIENTS

¼ medium avocado, mashed

1 slice whole-grain bread, toasted

2 teaspoons everything bagel seasoning

Pinch of flaky sea salt (such as Maldon)

INSTRUCTIONS

Spread avocado on toast. Top with seasoning and salt.

Baked Banana-Nut Oatmeal Cups

INGREDIENTS

3 cups rolled oats (see Tip)

1 ½ cups low-fat milk

2 ripe bananas, mashed (about 3/4 cup)

⅓ cup packed brown sugar

2 large eggs, lightly beaten

1 teaspoon baking powder

1 teaspoon ground cinnamon

1 teaspoon vanilla extract

½ teaspoon salt

½ cup toasted chopped pecans

INSTRUCTIONS

Preheat oven to 375°F. Coat a muffin tin with cooking spray.

Combine oats, milk, bananas, brown sugar, eggs, baking powder, cinnamon, vanilla and salt in a large bowl. Fold in pecans. Divide the mixture among the muffin cups (about 1/3 cup each). Bake until a toothpick inserted in the center comes out clean, about 25 minutes. Cool in the pan for 10 minutes, then turn out onto a wire rack. Serve warm or at room temperature.

Pineapple Green Smoothie

INGREDIENTS

½ cup unsweetened almond milk

⅓ cup nonfat plain Greek yogurt

1 cup baby spinach

1 cup frozen banana slices (about 1 medium banana)

½ cup frozen pineapple chunks

1 tablespoon chia seeds

1-2 teaspoons pure maple syrup or honey (optional)

INSTRUCTIONS

Add almond milk and yogurt to a blender, then add spinach, banana, pineapple, chia seeds and sweetener (if using); blend until smooth.

Muesli with Raspberries

INGREDIENTS

⅓ cup muesli

1 cup raspberries

¾ cup low-fat milk

INSTRUCTIONS

Top muesli with raspberries and serve with milk.

CHAPTER VI
NOURISHING LUNCH RECIPES FOR GALLSTONE PREVENTION

Butternut squash and sweet potato soup

INGREDIENTS

1 tbsp olive oil

1 medium onion, peeled and roughly chopped

2 cloves garlic, peeled and crushed

1 tsp hot curry powder

300g sweet potato, peeled weight and diced

250g butternut squash, peeled and deseeded weight and diced

500ml vegetable stock using 2 reduced-salt stock cubes

500ml Alpro Soya No Sugars alternative to milk

A small handful of basil leaves – torn

100g Alpro Plain No Sugars alternative to yogurt

INSTRUCTIONS time: 15 minutes

Cooking time: 20 minutes

Serves: 4

Nutrition: Per serving

Energy

199 KcalFat

6.6gSaturates

1.3gSugars

10.2gSalt

1.71g

This soup is really delicious either hot or cold, the hit of curry powder enhances the flavours of the sweet potato and the butternut squash. Contains 2 of you 5-a-day.

INSTRUCTIONS

Heat oil in large saucepan, add onion cook over medium heat until soft and translucent. Add the crushed garlic and curry powder and cook a further minute stirring.

Add sweet potato and butternut squash pieces, stir and cook for 2 minutes.

Add stock and Alpro Soya No Sugars, bring to the boil and reduce to a simmer for 20 minutes or until the sweet potato is cooked.

Allow to cool for a few minutes before pouring into a blender or a food processor with the basil leaves. Blend the mixture until smooth.

Serve soup hot or cold with a swirl of Alpro Plain No Sugars alternative to yogurt

Crunchy nachos with avocado dip

INGREDIENTS

For the avocado dip

2 ripe avocados

A handful of coriander, leaves only roughly chopped

1 lime, half the zest and half to all the juice

200g Alpro Greek Style Plain alternative to yogurt

¼ tsp cumin

Tiny pinch of salt

¼ tsp black pepper

2 fresh red chillies

For the nachos

4 wholewheat wraps

Serve with

10 cherry tomatoes, halved

2 spring onions, chopped

2 sweet peppers, sliced

INSTRUCTIONS

Preheat the oven to 200°C/180°C Fan/Gas mark 6.

For the dip: Peel the avocado, remove the stone and place the flesh into a bowl. Add the chopped coriander leaves, the zest and juice from one half of the lime and mash it all up using a potato masher or a fork. Add the Alpro Greek Style Plain, cumin, tiny pinch of salt and the black pepper and mix well until it's smooth. Finely chop the chillies, remove the seeds if you don't want it too spicy, and add these to the mix and stir well. Taste and add more lime juice if needed.

For the nachos: Cut each wrap into 8 triangular slices, spread them out on a baking tray. Bake in the preheated oven for 15 minutes, turning them over after 8 minutes until they're crispy and golden.

Serve the dip with the warm nachos, tomato halves, spring onions and pepper slices.

Carrot and Coriander Soup

INGREDIENTS

1 tablespoon sunflower or rapeseed oil

1 clove garlic, crushed

1 onion, chopped

2 medium carrots, grated

2 celery sticks, chopped

2 tomatoes, chopped

600mls low-salt vegetable stock

300mls orange juice

3 tablespoons freshly chopped coriander

freshly ground black pepper to season

INSTRUCTIONS

Heat the oil, add the garlic, onion, carrot, celery and tomatoes and cook for a few minutes until softened.

Add the stock, season and simmer for 20-25 minutes.

Add the coriander and orange juice.

Pulse in a blender, reheat, check the seasoning and serve.

Serve with chunks of wholegrain bread

Recipe Tip

Reduce salt further by using homemade vegetable stock or by using a low salt stock cube

Tomato Watercress Bruschetta

INGREDIENTS

1 wholegrain baguette

14 mini tomatoes, chopped

2 large handfuls of watercress, chopped roughly

2 sticks of spring onion, chopped

Small handful of oregano leaves, chopped

2 tsp lemon juice or balsamic vinegar

3 tbsp olive oil

60g pistachios, chopped roughly

Ground black pepper

INSTRUCTIONS

Combine the tomatoes, watercress, oregano and spring onions in a bowl, adding the lemon juice or balsamic vinegar and olive oil and toss together to combine.

Then add the pistachios and sprinkle some black pepper and toss again.

Diagonally slice the baguette into thin slices and toast. Top the toasts with a spoonful of the salad mixture and serve.

Falafel with aubergine dip

INGREDIENTS

Dip

40 gram Flora ProActiv Buttery

1 aubergine

2 tbsp olive oil

1 red bell pepper

2 garlic cloves crushed

1 pinch paprika

1/2 tsp ground cumin

2 tbsp fresh parsley chopped

4 pitta bread to serve

Falafel

400g tinned chickpeas drained

1 small onion finely chopped

1 clove garlic crushed

1 tsp ground cumin

1 tsp ground coriander

1 tbsp dried mixed herbs

1 tbsp flour

1 tbsp olive oil

INSTRUCTIONS

Preheat oven to 200°C/180°C Fan/Gas mark 6.

For the aubergine dip, cut the aubergine in half lengthways, place on baking sheet and brush with oil. Roast in oven for 25 to 30 minutes.

Grill the pepper until skin has blackened. Cool and then peel off skin. Remove seeds and finely chop flesh. Place in a bowl with garlic, Flora ProActiv Buttery spread, spices and herbs.

Spoon out aubergine flesh, chop finely and add to bowl. Mix well and season to taste.

For the falafel, place all ingredients except for oil in a food processor and blend until smooth or the texture you prefer. Form the mix into small balls and flatten slightly.

Brush with the oil and bake in oven for 15 to 20 minutes.

Serve both the aubergine and falafel with salad, in pitta breads or with crudités. Both can be kept in the fridge for 2 to 3 days.

Mediterranean Chicken Bagel

INGREDIENTS

1 seeded bagel

10g Flora ProActiv Light

1 garlic clove, cut in half

50g cooked chicken breast

1 sundried tomato, chopped into small pieces

10g kalamata olives, quartered

1 small tomato, sliced

A handful of rocket

Ground black pepper

Dried oregano to taste

INSTRUCTIONS

Toast the bagel

When it is toasted, rub the cut side of the garlic clove over both sides of the bagel

Spread the bagel with Flora ProActiv Light

Next layer up your bagel, starting with the chicken slices, followed by the sundried tomato and olives pieces, slices of tomato and rocket leaves

Season to taste with black pepper and sprinkle over some oregano

Butter Bean and Sundried Tomato Dip

INGREDIENTS

1 tin of butter beans (400g)

100g sundried tomatoes

1 clove garlic

1 tsp oregano

20g Flora ProActiv Light

1 tbsp tahini

2 tsp lemon juice

4 tbsp water

Freshly ground black pepper

To serve

1 carrot, chopped into batons

4 pitta breads

20g Flora ProActiv Light

INSTRUCTIONS

Place all the dip ingredients into a mini blender and blend until smooth.

Toast the pittas, slice open and spread inside the pittas with the Flora ProActiv. Cut into triangles.

Serve the dip with the pitta triangles and carrot sticks.

Veggie Burgers

INGREDIENTS

1 tsp olive oil

1 red onion, chopped

2 cloves garlic

1 carrot, grated

1 large flat mushroom (approx. 65g), chopped

1 tsp paprika

½ tsp cumin

Ground black pepper

½ can kidney beans, drained (120g)

½ can butter beans, drained (120g)

1 slice seeded bread, torn into pieces

4 small brioche burger buns

40g Flora ProActiv Light

Lettuce leaves

2 small tomatoes

4 tbsp Light mayonnaise

INSTRUCTIONS

Preheat the oven to 220°C/200°C Fan/Gas mark 7.

Heat olive oil in a large frying pan and fry onion over a medium heat for about three minutes.

Add the carrot, mushrooms and garlic and cook for another five minutes.

Add the spices and black pepper and cook for another minute. Remove from the heat.

Add about three quarters of the beans, the mushroom mixture and the bread to a food processor and pulse until the mixture starts to come together. Add the remaining beans and pulse briefly so some of the beans are still whole.

Shape the mixture into 4 burger shapes.

Place onto a baking tray lined with baking parchment.

Cook for 20-25 minutes until lightly browned and hot all the way through.

Serve with a toasted roll spread with Flora ProActiv Light, and topped with slices of tomato, lettuce and light mayonnaise.

Shakshuka with Garlic Pittas

INGREDIENTS

Shakshuka

1 tbsp vegetable oil

1 red onion

1 red pepper

1 yellow pepper

1.5 tsp cumin

1.5 tsp paprika

1 tsp chilli powder

2 cloves garlic, crushed

1 can chopped tomatoes

2 tbsp tomato puree

½ can chickpeas, drained

4 medium eggs

Freshly ground black pepper

A handful fresh parsley, chopped

Garlic Pittas

4 wholemeal pita bread

1-2 cloves garlic, crushed

40g ProActiv Light

Freshly ground black pepper

INSTRUCTIONS

Roughly chop the onion and peppers

In a large frying pan or wok, heat the vegetable oil over a medium heat. Fry the onion for a few minutes until starting to soften, then add the peppers for another five minutes

Add the garlic and spices and cook for another minute or two until fragrant

Add the tomatoes, tomato puree and chickpeas. Simmer for about 15 minutes until the sauce thickens

While the sauce is simmering, prepare the garlic pittas. Preheat oven to 200°C/180°C Fan/Gas mark 6. Mix the ProActiv Light with one-two cloves of crushed garlic (depending on how garlicy you like it!) and black pepper. Set aside

When the sauce has reduced, use a wooden spoon to make four wells in the tomato sauce. Crack an egg into each as quickly as you can

Cover the pan with a lid and cook for 5-10 minutes depending on how you like your eggs

Put the pitta breads into the oven on a baking tray while the eggs are cooking, and cook for 8 minutes

Check the egg whites are cooked and yolks are to your liking and take off the heat. Season with black pepper and plenty of fresh parsley

Spread the garlic ProActiv mix onto the hot pittas and serve with the shakshuka

Mediterranean Soup

INGREDIENTS

1 onion, finely chopped

1 clove garlic, crushed

1 tbsp olive oil

1 bell pepper (red or yellow), diced

2 courgettes, diced

1 tsp paprika

1 tsp fresh rosemary, chopped

1 tsp Balsamic vinegar

400g can chopped or pureed tomatoes

1-litre vegetable stock made from 2 low salt stock cubes

1 tbsp Tomato puree

1 sprig fresh flat-leaf parsley (optional)

Freshly ground pepper

INSTRUCTIONS

Heat the oil in a pan and gently cook the onion and garlic for 5 minutes without colouring.

Set aside 1 tbsp of diced pepper then add the remainder of the pepper along with the courgettes, paprika, rosemary to the pan and cook for a few minutes.

Add the balsamic vinegar, after 2 minutes add the tomatoes and stock and bring to the boil.

Gently simmer until the vegetables are cooked through and tender, about 10 minutes.

Finally, stir in the tomato paste. Either leave the soup as a rustic, chunky vegetable broth or use a handheld blender to blend until smooth.

Season with fresh ground pepper and serve topped with the reserved diced pepper and a sprig of parsley.

CHAPTER VII

NOURISHING DINNER RECIPES FOR GALLSTONE PREVENTION

Savory Chicken kebabs with garlic sauce and pickles

INGREDIENTS

For the marinade

2 x cloves of garlic, peeled and chopped

1 tbsp of olive oil

A pinch of smoked paprika

White pepper

2 x chicken breasts cut into 2cm strips

For the garlic sauce

150g 0% fat Greek yoghurt

1 clove of garlic, peeled and finely chopped

1 tbsp chopped flat-leaf parsley

Squeeze of lemon juice

For the wrap

2 large wholemeal wraps

4 leaves of lettuce

2 small vine tomatoes, quartered

½ small red onion, finely sliced

1 small pickled gherkin, finely sliced

A dash of tabasco

INSTRUCTIONS

To make the marinade, stir together the garlic, oil, paprika and white pepper. Add the chicken and mix thoroughly. Cover and refrigerate for at least 12 hours.

Preheat the oven to 190C (170C Fan), Gas Mark 5.

To make the garlic sauce, mix together the yoghurt, garlic, parsley and lemon juice. If it's easier, this can be made a day in advance.

Thread the chicken pieces on to two wooden skewers (if you soak the skewers before using them, they will not burn). Rest these onto a baking tray and place in the oven and cook for 15 minutes, or until cooked through. Remove the chicken from the skewers.

Lay the wraps on two plates and spread over the garlic sauce. Roll each wrap into a cone shape. Stuff with the lettuce, chicken, tomatoes, red onion, pickled gherkin and finally a dash of Tabasco. Serve immediately.

Savory Veggie Lasagne

INGREDIENTS

500g mushrooms

2 courgettes

1 tbsp olive oil

2 shallots, finely chopped

1 clove garlic, crushed

24 to 28 cherry tomatoes, halved

Half a bunch fresh parsley, finely chopped

1 tsp Herbs de Provence

Salt & pepper

50g vegetable spread e.g. olive, sunflower

50g plain flour

600ml of Alpro Soya Unsweetened alternative to milk

12 sheets of lasagne

A pinch grated nutmeg

INSTRUCTIONS

Preheat the oven to 200°C/180°C Fan/Gas mark 6.

Slice the mushrooms and courgettes. Sauté the shallots, garlic and mushrooms in 1 tablespoon of olive oil for 5 minutes. Add the sliced courgettes, halved cherry tomatoes and the chopped parsley and allow to simmer for 3 minutes. Add the Herbs de Provence, a pinch of salt and a good pinch of ground pepper.

For the bechamel sauce: Over a medium to high heat, melt the vegetable spread in a saucepan and sprinkle in the flour while stirring continuously for 2-3 minutes until you obtain a smooth mixture and it all comes together. Remove the pan from the heat and pour in a little of the Alpro Soya Unsweetened at time, stirring well after each addition to produce a smooth paste. Once all the Alpro Soya Unsweetened has been incorporated, place the pan back on the heat and bring to a simmer, stirring continuously and allow to simmer and thicken for 1-2 minutes. Stir and bring to a simmer. Allow it to simmer until the desired thickness is achieved. Remove from the heat, add a small pinch of salt, a good pinch of ground pepper and a good pinch of grated nutmeg – stir well.

Assemble the lasagne in your baking dish: cover the base of the baking dish with one third of the vegetables, cover with a layer of lasagne sheets followed by one third of the bechamel sauce. Repeat twice more ending with a layer of bechamel sauce.

Place in the preheated oven and bake for 40 to 45 minutes.

Tuna Pasta Bake

INGREDIENTS

400g wholemeal pasta shapes (we used Fusilli)

2x 160g tins tuna in water, drained

100g of spinach

1 can sweetcorn, drained

75g wholemeal breadcrumbs

1 x 500ml jar of tomato sauce

100g 10% fat mozzarella cheese, grated or cut into small pieces

Black pepper

INSTRUCTIONS

Warm the oven to 200C (180C for a fan oven).

Cook the pasta in a large pan (following the pack instructions) until cooked but still firm - "al dente".

Add the spinach to the pan of pasta for the last minute and allow to wilt.

Drain and transfer the pasta and spinach to a large baking dish.

Mix in the tuna, sweetcorn and tomato sauce and season with black pepper.

Top with the mozzarella and finally with the breadcrumbs.

Bake for at least 30 minutes or until bubbling.

Serve.

Recipe Tip

Try using other vegetables favourites including peas, mixed vegetables, broccoli florets, asparagus tips, mushrooms or bell peppers

Plaice goujons with a California Walnut Crust

INGREDIENTS

90g California walnuts, toasted

Small bunch of parsley

Finely-grated zest of 1 lemon

40g panko bread crumbs

A pinch black pepper

4 level tbsp light mayonnaise

2 tsp Dijon mustard

1/2 tbsp water

300g plaice, skinned and cut into fingers

Rapeseed oil spray

Baby spinach leaves and lemon wedges to serve (optional)

INSTRUCTIONS

Preheat the oven to 180°C.

Place the walnuts, parsley and lemon zest into a food processor and blitz to a fine crumb. Mix with the panko bread crumbs and pepper, and place on a dinner plate.

Mix together the mayonnaise and Dijon, then loosen with the water to form a good dipping consistency.

Dip the plaice fingers into the mayonnaise mix and then roll in the breadcrumb mixture to coat.

Place on a flat baking tray lined with parchment which has been spritzed with 4-5 sprays of rapeseed oil. Drizzle the goujons with a little oil and place in the oven for 15- 20 minutes (or until cooked through and crispy golden on the outside).

Serve on a bed of baby spinach with lemon wedges to the side.

Prawn and Vegetable Curry

INGREDIENTS

For the curry:

4 cloves garlic

1 onion

1 tbsp olive oil

1 apple, grated

2½ tbsp curry powder

1 tsp garam masala

½ tsp turmeric

400g chopped tomatoes, tinned

½ red chilli, chopped finely

200ml boiling water

2 tsp sweetener

110g (7 tbsp) tinned chickpeas, drained and rinsed

200g frozen prawns

50ml soya milk

Few coriander leaves

For the rice:

265g basmati rice / 1 ½ cups

400ml boiled water

INSTRUCTIONS

Measure and pour out the basmati rice, cover with the boiled water and cook according to packet instructions.

Cook the garlic and onion in olive oil over a medium heat until golden. Add the curry powder, garam masala and turmeric and cook for a further minute. Add in the grated apple, chopped tomatoes and red chilli and stir to combine then add 200ml of water and stir again. Bring up to the simmer and cook for a further 2 minutes.

Add the chickpeas and frozen prawns and cook until they soften and are hot all the way through. Once hot, stir in the sweetener and soya milk.

Serve the rice and curry in a bowl and garnish with coriander leaves.

Savory Chinese Chicken Curry

INGREDIENTS

4 skinless chicken breasts, cut into chunks

2 tsp cornflour

1 onion, diced

100g mushrooms, sliced

2 tbsp rapeseed oil

1 garlic clove, crushed

2 tsp curry powder

1 tsp turmeric

½ tsp ground ginger

Pinch sugar

400ml chicken stock, reduced salt

1 tsp soy sauce, reduced salt

Handful frozen peas

INSTRUCTIONS

Toss the chicken pieces in the cornflour and season well. Set them aside.

Fry the onion in half of the oil in a frying pan or wok on a low to medium heat, until it softens – about 5-6 minutes. Then add the garlic and cook for a minute. Stir in the spices and sugar and cook for another minute, then add the stock and soy sauce, bring to a simmer and cook for 20 minutes. Tip everything into a blender and blitz until smooth.

Wipe out the pan and fry the chicken in the remaining oil until it is browned all over. Add the mushrooms and fry for a couple of minutes. Tip the sauce back into the pan and bring everything to a simmer, stir in the peas and cook for 5 minutes or until the chicken is cooked through. Add a little water if you need to thin the sauce.

Serve with rice.

Sardines and Pasta

INGREDIENTS

Rapeseed Oil spray

1 onion, finely diced

3 fresh sardines, cleaned, scaled, filleted and cut into bite sized chunks (or a can of sardines or 2-3 smoked fillets of mackerel skin removed)

2 tbsp tomato puree

1 (approximately 100g) roasted red pepper – roughly sliced

6 cherry or baby plum tomatoes, sliced into quarters

1 tbsp currants

1/2 tbsp sun-dried tomato puree

½ bag fresh pasta (spaghetti or pasta shapes)

1 tbsp toasted pine nuts

Fennel fronds

INSTRUCTIONS

Heat a large frying pan over a medium heat and spritz 4 times with rapeseed oil spray. Add the onion and cook for a few minutes, without colour and until softened.

Add the sardine pieces, tomato puree and a ladle of water. Stir and cook gently for a few minutes.

Add the toasted pine nuts, currants, tomatoes and red pepper, cook for a further 10-15 minutes.

Meanwhile cook the fresh pasta in boiling water for about 6 minutes, until tender but still firm (al dente).

Add the cooked pasta to the sardine mix, season, stir and dish up in warm bowls garnished with fennel.

Serve with fresh Italian bread and a green side salad.

Sea Bass with a Vegetable Ensemble

INGREDIENTS

For the fish:

4 sea bass fillets (1 fillet = 110g)

2 garlic cloves, finely chopped

1 onion, finely chopped

100ml white wine

1 tbsp low fat spread

A small handful of parsley, finely chopped

Few leaves of curly-leaf parsley, to decorate

½ lemon, juiced, and 4 slices to decorate

Ground pepper

For the stuffed open mushroom:

4 large Portobello mushrooms

4 tbsp wholemeal breadcrumbs

20g pistachios, chopped

2 tbsp grated reduced-fat mozzarella

2 tbsp grated reduced-fat cheddar cheese

1 tsp olive oil + rapeseed oil spray to spritz the foil

A small handful of parsley, finely chopped

Ground pepper

250g cherry tomatoes, on the vine

For the sweet potato:

650g sweet potatoes (or 4 medium sized sweet potatoes), diced

Rapeseed oil spray

1 tbsp finely chopped fresh rosemary (or 1.5 tsp dried rosemary)

Ground pepper

INSTRUCTIONS

Preheat the oven to 180°C. Prepare two baking trays, line both with foil and spritz one with rapeseed oil spray. Finely chop the garlic cloves and onion and leave aside. Then prepare the sweet potato by peeling the skin, cutting them into cubes and placing them on the non-greased tray. Spritz the sweet potatoes with rapeseed oil spray and place them in the oven for 25 minutes.

In the meantime, in a small bowl, combine the breadcrumbs, cheese, chopped pistachios, parsley and stir with a teaspoon of olive oil and some ground pepper. Wipe the outside of the mushrooms with dry fingers (do not rinse under water as this makes the mushrooms soggy), place on the other greased baking tray with the stalks facing up. Fill the mushrooms with the breadcrumb and pistachio mixture and place in the oven for 15 minutes. After the mushrooms have been in the oven of 15 minutes, place the tomatoes in the oven next to them.

Over a medium heat, melt half a tablespoon of low fat spread in a frying pan and cook the onions and garlic until brown and leave aside in a dish. Using the other half of the low fat spread, cook the sea bass fillets in a non stick pan, skin side down for 3 minutes. Add the squeezed lemon juice and white wine and let them cook for another few minutes.

Pour the garlic and onions back into the surrounding juice, and add the chopped parsley. Turn over the fillets and cook for another 2 minutes.

Place all the components on a plate, and decorate the sea bass with a lemon slice and few whole leaves of parsley.

Savory Prawn skewers with flatbreads

INGREDIENTS

1 tbsp garam masala

¼ tsp ground turmeric

150g low-fat natural yogurt

200g raw peeled king prawns

2-3 inch piece cucumber, seeds removed

10g fresh mint (a handful) roughly chopped or 1 tbsp from a jar of mint sauce

1 lime

25g baby leaf salad

2 chapattis or wraps, cooked without fat

INSTRUCTIONS

If using wooden skewers pre-soak these to stop them burning.

Mix together the garam marsala, turmeric and half the yogurt. Add the prawns and mix to coat them with the yogurt mixture. Thread onto 6 skewers. Set aside.

Grate the cucumber, squeezing out any excess liquid. Mix with the remaining yogurt, chopped mint and a squeeze of lime juice, to taste. Place in a serving bowl.

Grill or barbeque the skewers for 3 minutes on each side until cooked through.

Pile the salad leaves onto the flat breads and top with the skewers. Serve with the mint and cucumber yogurt and lime wedges.

Savory Roasted tomato and broccoli pasta

INGREDIENTS

4 garlic cloves, peeled

400g cherry tomatoes

Few sprigs thyme

1 tbsp olive oil

300g spaghetti or other shaped pasta, wholemeal if possible

400g tenderstem broccoli, broken into up into florets

50g pine nuts

40g cashew nuts

40g almonds

2 tbsp olive oil

1 onion, finely chopped

½ tsp chilli flakes

5 tbsp plain flour

1L Alpro Oat Unsweetened drink

Pinch salt and pepper

½-1 lemon, juice

Large bunch of fresh basil leaves

1 tbsp extra Virgin Olive Oil

INSTRUCTIONS

Preheat the oven to 200°C/180°C Fan/Gas mark 6.

Put the whole peeled garlic cloves and whole cherry tomatoes on a baking tray. Add the sprigs of thyme, drizzle with the tablespoon of olive oil and mix well to evenly coat the tomatoes and garlic. Place in the preheated oven and roast for 25-30 minutes until the tomatoes have blistered and a little coloured, remove from the oven and set aside. Once cooled, remove the garlic cloves and finely chop or mash.

Meanwhile, bring a large pan of water to the boil and cook the pasta to pack instructions. Add the broccoli florets for the last 3 minutes of cooking time, then drain and set aside.

In a dry non-stick pan on medium to high heat, quickly toast the pine nuts until golden, remove from the heat and pour into a container to cool. Place the pan back on the heat and add the cashews and almonds and toast until lightly golden, remove from the heat, pour into a container to cool before roughly chopping and mixing with the pine nuts.

In a large deep saucepan, heat 2 tbsp of oil over a medium heat and add the onion. Gently fry for 5-8 minutes until softened and a little coloured. Add the chilli flakes and flour and fry for a few minutes until bubbling.

Remove from the heat, add the chopped or mashed roasted garlic and stir well. Gradually incorporate the Alpro Oat Unsweetened drink by adding just a little at a time and stirring well after each addition to combine to a smooth paste. Once all the Alpro Oat Unsweetened has been incorporated, place the pan back onto a medium heat and stirring continuously bring to a simmer and cook for a couple of minutes until the sauce is thick. Season with a small pinch salt, some ground pepper and a squeeze of lemon.

Assemble your dish. Toss the cooked spaghetti and broccoli through the bechamel sauce. Top with the roasted tomatoes, toasted nuts, a handful of fresh basil and drizzle with the 1 tbsp olive oil.

Spanish Fish Stew

INGREDIENTS

3 tbsp olive oil

1 white onion

2 fennel bulbs

1 red chilli

400g chopped tomatoes

100ml fish stock

150ml white wine

500g mussels

650g firm white fish eg cod, monkfish cut into bite-size pieces

2 cloves of garlic

50g chorizo

1½ tsp sweet paprika

1 tsp saffron

3 bay leaves

INSTRUCTIONS

Heat the oil in a frying pan and add the onion, fennel, chorizo, chilli and garlic and saute for 3 minutes.

Add the paprika, saffron, bay leaves and tomatoes, and leave until reduced to a sauce of a thick consistency.

Meanwhile, scrub the mussels and pull away any stringy beards. Any that are open should be tapped sharply on the worktop – if they don't close after a few seconds, discard them.

Add the fish stock and white wine to the pot and bring to a gentle simmer. Stir the chunks of fish very gently into the stew. Bring back to the simmer, then cover and cook gently for 3 mins.

Scatter over the mussels, recover and let them cook until they have opened (about 2 minutes). The chunks of fish should flake easily when cooked through and the mussels should have opened wide, throw away any that do not open.

Remove the bay leaves and serve.

Savory Spicy Burgers

INGREDIENTS

450g (1 lb) minced chicken

1 onion, grated

2 garlic cloves, crushed

1 teaspoon paprika

INSTRUCTIONS

Preheat the grill to medium.

Mix all the ingredients together.

Shape the mixture into 8 burgers.

Grill under medium heat for 4-5 minutes each side or until the meat is completely cooked through.

Serve with salad or in wholemeal rolls.

CHAPTER VIII
NOURISHING MAIN DISH RECIPES FOR GALLSTONE PREVENTION

Chipotle Black Bean Chili

INGREDIENTS

3 cups dried black beans (turtle beans)

2 tablespoons olive oil

1 large green bell pepper, cored, seeded, finely chopped (about 2 cups)

2 large onions, finely chopped (about 6 cups)

8 cloves garlic, finely minced (about 1/3 cup)

2 large carrots finely chopped (about 2 cups)

1 canned chipotle pepper in adobo sauce, seeds discarded, finely chopped

1 tablespoon ground cumin

2 tablespoons dried oregano leaves

1 28-ounce can low-sodium crushed or diced tomatoes

¼ cups white vinegar

1 teaspoon pepper

Suggested garnish: finely chopped red or green onion or cilantro with a dollop of nonfat sour cream or Greek yogurt.

INSTRUCTIONS

Rinse beans 2 or 3 times. Then, place in a very large pot, add half each of the green pepper and garlic and cover with 3 quarts of hot water. Cover the pot and bring to a gentle boil, then simmer for 90 minutes or until beans are tender, but still firm. This cooking method replaces soaking the beans overnight.

Place olive oil in another large skillet and sauté remaining green pepper, garlic, onions, and carrots until very tender, 20-30 minutes.

Add cumin, oregano, tomatoes, vinegar and chipotle to sautéed vegetables and simmer 10 more minutes.

Add vegetables to the beans and cook over medium-low heat, stirring often, until beans can be mashed with a spoon, 10-20 minutes.

Use a blender or food processor to puree 3-4 cups of chili and add back into pot, mixing it all together. Dish up, garnish, and serve.

Per 1 cup serving: 256 calories, 13g protein, 47g carbohydrate, 3g fat, 1g sat fat, 2g mono fat, 1mg cholesterol, 16g fiber, 128mg sodium.

Okra and Octopus Pasta Bowl

INGREDIENTS

5 medium sized okra pods

1 teaspoon olive oil

1 spring onion, chopped from bulb to end of green stalk

1 can of octopus parts in oil

1 tablespoon of undiluted tomato paste

2 tablespoons of warm water

1 tablespoon balsamic vinegar

oregano and basil to taste

INSTRUCTIONS

To keep it simple, okra is actually great for people! It has no fat or cholesterol, it does have potassium, and vitamin a in spades. There's no sodium, so great for those of us with high blood pressure, and that dreaded stickiness serves to thicken stews like gumbo. How bad can anything in gumbo really be? People in the Southern part of the US feature okra in so many recipes, that it's shameful NOT to eat it. Who could resist something called Fried Pecan Okra? And if you're still not sure, WikiHow even has a full page with videos on how to prepare okra.

Wash and trim a handful of okra pods. Cut of stem ends.

Pour a teaspoonful of olive oil into a skillet and heat.

Add chopped fresh spring onion, garlic, oregano, basil, and a can of chopped octopus. Saute for a few minutes and then add a cupful of halved cherry tomatoes. Cook for a few minutes to blend flavors

add half of a can of tomato paste diluted with a few tablespoons of warm water. Add the diluted paste to the skillet and stir. If it's too thick add water to loosen it up.

Add a brimming tablespoon of balsamic vinegar, stir, and then cover. Simmer on low heat.

Boil up some pasta to an al dente texture. Heap pasta in a bowl, then ladle on the sauce. Sprinkle on a little parmesan and enjoy with a hearty glass of red wine.

Chicken Biryani

INGREDIENTS

2.5 pounds chicken

1.5 pounds White boiled rice

1 cup water

1 cup cooking oil

1 teaspoon garlic and ginger paste

1/2 teaspoon salt

2 teaspoons Red pepper

4 teaspoons Biryani masala

2 bay leafs

2 chopped red onions

INSTRUCTIONS

Cooking instructions for Red onions 1. Take a wok and add half cup of oil over medium-high heat 2. Add half cup of chopped onions in heated oil 3. Cook them until dark brown color 4. Put Out them in a bowl after fry

Cooking instructions for chicken 1. Put half cup of in a large wok over medium-high heat 2. Now add 4tb spoon biryani masala and garlic paste in oil 3.Add salt, red, and black pepper 4.Add bay leaf and half cup of water and cook them for 5 to 10 minutes 5.Now add chicken and half cup of water and mix these ingredients and cook them well 20 minutes 6. During cooking of chicken make normal gravy for biryani recipe

Cooking instructions for Biryani 1. After cooking the chicken with gravy Now Add boiled rice on chicken 2. Cover them for 10 minutes over Low-medium heat 4. After 10 minutes Now mix them well that all ingredients mix with each other 5. You can also add some pickle for spicy taste and mix with biryani

You can serve this recipe with raita and salad and for more taste, you can add some pickle. People of South Asian countries like to eat this recipe with spicy taste and other ingredients. In Hyderabadi biryani recipe, fried potatoes are used with chicken for extra flavor. for more you can check my food blog theamazingrecipes.com

Chicken Biryani Recipe full Nutritional Information Chicken biryani is full of healthy ingredients that include chicken and boiled rice. These ingredients are full of healthy calories, vitamins, and proteins. Here, we will tell you about the nutrition information of this recipe with quantity. Total Calories 2,080 Sodium 760 mg Total Fats 68 g Potassium 2,147 mg Saturated 38 g Total Carbs 232 g Polyunsaturated 3 g Dietary Fiber 22 g Monounsaturated 16 g Sugar 34 g Trans 0 g Protein 137 g Cholesterol 399 mg Vitamin A 73% Calcium 69% Vitamin C 8% Iron 75%

Black Beans and Rice

INGREDIENTS

1 teaspoon olive oil

1 onion, chopped

2 cloves garlic, minced

¾ cup uncooked white rice

1 ½ cups low sodium, low fat vegetable broth

3 ½ cups canned black beans, drained

1 teaspoon ground cumin

¼ teaspoon cayenne pepper

INSTRUCTIONS

Heat oil in a saucepan over medium-high heat. Add onion and garlic; cook and stir until onion has softened, about 4 minutes. Stir in rice to coat; cook and stir for 2 minutes.

Add vegetable broth and bring to a boil. Cover, reduce to a simmer, and cook until liquid is absorbed, about 20 minutes.

Stir in beans, cumin, and cayenne; cook until beans are warmed through.

Pesto Pasta with Chicken

INGREDIENTS

1 (16 ounce) package bow tie pasta

1 teaspoon olive oil

2 cloves garlic, minced

2 skinless, boneless chicken breasts, cut into bite-sized pieces

1 pinch crushed red pepper flakes, or to taste

½ cup pesto sauce

⅓ cup oil-packed sun-dried tomatoes, drained and cut into strips

INSTRUCTIONS

Gather all ingredients.

Bring a large pot of lightly salted water to a boil. Add pasta and cook until al dente, 8 to 10 minutes; drain.

Heat oil in a large skillet over medium heat. Sauté garlic until tender.

Stir in chicken and season with red pepper flakes. Cook until chicken is golden and cooked through.

Combine pasta, chicken, pesto, and sun-dried tomatoes in a large bowl; toss to coat evenly.

CHAPTER VIII

NOURISHING SOUP RECIPES FOR GALLSTONE PREVENTION

Red Lentil Dhal Soup with Indian Spiced Broccoli

INGREDIENTS

For the Dhal

2 tbsp vegetable oil

1 onion, finely chopped

1 garlic clove, crushed or grated

1 tsp grated fresh ginger

1 red chilli, deseeded and finely chopped

1 tsp ground turmeric

1 tsp garam masala

200g red split lentils

1.3L reduced salt vegetable stock

½ lemon, juiced

3 x 67.5ml bottles Benecol Original Yogurt drinks

For the broccoli

150g long-stemmed broccoli, cut into large pieces

1 tsp vegetable oil

1 tsp mustard seeds

1 tsp cumin seeds

1 tsp coriander seeds

1 tsp dried red chilli flakes

INSTRUCTIONS

Preheat your oven to 180°C/1600C Fan/Gas 4.

Heat the vegetable oil in a pan over medium-high heat and add the onion. Cook the onion, stirring from time to time, for 5-8 minutes until it is soft. Add the garlic, ginger and red chilli, and cook for 1 minute before adding the turmeric and garam masala and cooking for another 30 seconds to release the aromas. Stir in the lentils. Pour in the stock, reduce the heat and gently simmer for 20 minutes until the lentils start to break down.

While the lentils cook, make the spicy broccoli. Place the broccoli in an oven proof dish, drizzle with vegetable oil and toss to combine. Sprinkle with the mustard seeds, cumin seeds, coriander seeds and chilli and bake in the oven for 15 minutes until the broccoli is cooked through and crispy on the edges.

Return to the lentil soup, add the Benecol Original Yogurt drinks, stir well, and bring back up to temperature, do not boil. Stir through the lemon juice.

To serve: divide the soup between 4 bowls and top with the broccoli and serve with wholemeal rolls

This recipe includes 1.5g plant stanol ester per serving*

*This recipe provides 1.5g of plant stanol esters per serving. Plant stanol ester has been shown to lower cholesterol in as little as 2-3 weeks. High cholesterol is a risk factor in the development of coronary heart disease. The beneficial effect has been shown with a daily intake of 1.5-3.0g plant stanols, as part, of a healthy diet and lifestyle.

Pea and Edamame Soup

INGREDIENTS

1 tbsp olive oil

200g frozen soya beans (also called edamame beans)

200g frozen peas

500ml hot reduced salt vegetable stock

1 onion, chopped

1 small bunch basil leaves

1 handful (50g) watercress

300ml Alpro Soya No Sugars alternative to milk

INSTRUCTIONS

Heat the oil in a saucepan. Add the onion and fry for 3 minutes. Add the frozen soya beans, frozen peas, vegetable stock and stir well. Bring to the boil and simmer for five minutes.

Add the basil and watercress and Alpro Soya No Sugars and warm through for 2-3 minutes. Taking care, blend with a hand blender until smooth and creamy. Season with black pepper. Serve warm with wholemeal bread.

Spiced Lentil and Carrot Soup

INGREDIENTS

2 tablespoons rapeseed oil

1 teaspoon cumin seeds

1 medium onion, finely sliced

2 cloves garlic, finely chopped

2 green chillies finely chopped

½ can tinned tomatoes

½ teaspoon turmeric

200g carrots, peeled and grated

50g split red lentils

1 litre low salt vegetable stock

Parsley sprigs to garnish

INSTRUCTIONS

Heat the oil in a heavy based saucepan, add the cumin seeds, onion, garlic and chillies and cook gently until onions slightly golden.

Add the tomatoes and turmeric, stirring well for a further few minutes.

Add the carrots and continue cooking gently for another few minutes.

Add the lentils, stir well and pour the vegetable stock and bring to boil. Lower the heat, cover and simmer gently for about 20 minutes or until lentils are just tender. Serve hot with parsley sprigs.

Mushroom and Hazelnut Broth

INGREDIENTS

2 tsp olive oil

150g chestnut mushrooms + 10g for a garnish

20 whole hazelnuts

250mls reduced salt vegetable stock

Black pepper

Chopped fresh parsley for garnish

INSTRUCTIONS

Clean and slice the mushrooms. Cook gently in a saucepan in the olive oil until soft, about 5-10 minutes. Reserve 3-4 slices for garnish.

Add the hazelnuts and stock to the pan and season with ground black pepper.

Simmer for 10-15 minutes.

Allow to cool and puree.

Reheat and serve garnished with sliced mushrooms and chopped parsley

Barley and Mushroom Chicken Soup

INGREDIENTS

1 tablespoon olive oil

1 medium onion, diced

1 cup red pepper, diced

4 cloves garlic, minced

2 cups mushrooms, bite-size pieces

2 cups broth from Slow-Cook Chicken or store-bought

6 cups water

1 cup cooked chicken, shredded

½ cups hulled or pearled barley

2 cups mixed greens (spinach, beet greens or swiss chard), chopped

½ teaspoons each salt, pepper and dried thyme

INSTRUCTIONS

Heat oil on medium heat in a large pot. Sauté onion, pepper, garlic and mushrooms until soft; about 5 minutes.

Add chicken broth and water to onion mixture; bring to a boil then reduce heat to medium low. Stir in chicken and barley.

Simmer until barley is tender; about 30 minutes for pearled barley, 60 minutes for hulled.

Stir in mixed greens and seasonings in final 10 minutes of cooking.

Per serving: 166 calories, 12g protein, 21g carbohydrate, 5g fat (1g sat, 3g mono/poly), 19mg cholesterol, 5g fiber, 291mg sodium

Seasoned Cook Make a double batch and freeze for a quick weeknight dinner. Mushrooms are high in vitamin D and beta-glucans, a fiber that lowers cholesterol Serve with arugula, avocado and orange salad.

Chunky Tomato Basil Sauce

INGREDIENTS

1 tablespoon olive oil

1 cup onion finely diced

2 cloves garlic, minced

1 15-ounce can diced tomatoes

¼ cups water or broth

INSTRUCTIONS

Heat olive oil over medium heat in pan, add onion and garlic. Sauté for 2-3 minutes or until onion is barely translucent.

Add tomatoes and basil, stir and bring to low boil for 3-5 minutes depending on desired thickness.

Per ½ cup serving: 65 calories, 2g protein, 8g carbohydrate, 4g fat, 1g sat fat, 3g mono fat, 0mg cholesterol, 2g fiber, 11mg sodium

Walk Away Slow-Cook Chicken

INGREDIENTS

1 whole chicken, 4-5 pounds

1 large onion

3 tablespoons combined of your favorite dried herbs/spices

INSTRUCTIONS

Rinse and dry chicken.

Roughly chop onion and place in bottom of slow-cooker.

Combine herbs and spices in a small bowl and gently rub on chicken.

Place chicken in slow-cooker on top of onions. Set on low for 3-8 hours depending on your appliance.

Before serving, drain the broth and save for soup.

Per 3.5 oz serving: 177 calories, 27g protein, 0 carbohydrates, 7g fat (2g sat, 4g mono/poly), 83mg cholesterol, 0g fiber, 70mg sodium

Seasoned Cook - For a savory bird, add ½ a lemon in the cavity and choose spices such as thyme, sage and basil. For a Latin flare, use chili powder, cayenne pepper, paprika and cumin as pictured here.

Cook Once, Eat Twice - Save leftover chicken and broth for soup.

Southern Fish Stew

INGREDIENTS

1 medium onion, sliced into thin strips

1 cup lima beans, canned or frozen

½ cups chicken or vegetable broth, low sodium

2 cups fresh or frozen okra

1 14.5 ounces can tomatoes with juice, diced or cut, stewed or with spices

1 teaspoon basil, oregano, thyme

1 pinch cayenne (optional for a little zing)

¾ pounds firm fish cut into edible chunks (snapper or cod are excellent)

INSTRUCTIONS

Spray nonstick pan with olive oil and sauté the onion over medium heat for a few minutes until wilted, but not brown.

Stir in lima beans and chicken broth. Simmer covered for 5 minutes.

Serve in bowls by itself or over a ½ cup serving of rice or polenta. Garnish with sliced black olives and chopped cilantro.

Per serving: 187 calories, 21 gm protein, 24 gm carbohydrate,1 gm fat, 0 gm sat, 0 gm mono, 31 mg cholesterol, 5 gm fiber, 320 mg sodium

THE SEASONED COOK You can substitute green bean, zucchini, kale, spinach or shredded cabbage for okra or lima beans. Keep it simple. Also, keep frozen or canned vegetables on hand to create this perfect simple supper if you are low on fresh ones. For an even more down home flavor, use smoked paprika.

CHAPTER IX
BEFORE YOU LEAVE, A FINAL WORD!

Following a diet aimed at preventing gallstones not only helps in avoiding the formation of these painful stones but also promotes overall digestive health and well-being. A high-fiber, low-fat diet can support a healthy weight, reduce the risk of other digestive issues, and contribute to long-term cardiovascular health. Additionally, moderate consumption of olive oil has been shown to lower cholesterol levels in the blood and gallbladder, further reducing the risk of gallstones. By maintaining a balanced diet and healthy lifestyle, you can enjoy improved digestion, reduced risk of gallstone complications, and better overall health.

www.ingramcontent.com/pod-product-compliance
Lightning Source LLC
Chambersburg PA
CBHW071831210526
45479CB00001B/78